YUMBOX

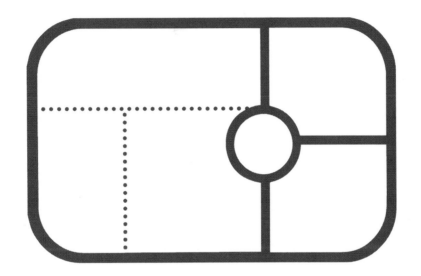

ORIGINAL, PANINO & TAPAS

Make it Happen Publishing Inc.

www.SylinaLunches.com
Send all inquires to sylina@sylinalunches.com

ISBN: 978-1-989116-41-8

Lunch Planning

WEEK OF:

MONDAY

SNACKS _____

_____

_____

TUESDAY

SNACKS _____

_____

_____

WEDNESDAY

SNACKS _____

_____

_____

THURSDAY

SNACKS _____

_____

_____

FRIDAY

SNACKS _____

_____

_____

NOTES

Lunch Planning

WEEK OF:

MONDAY

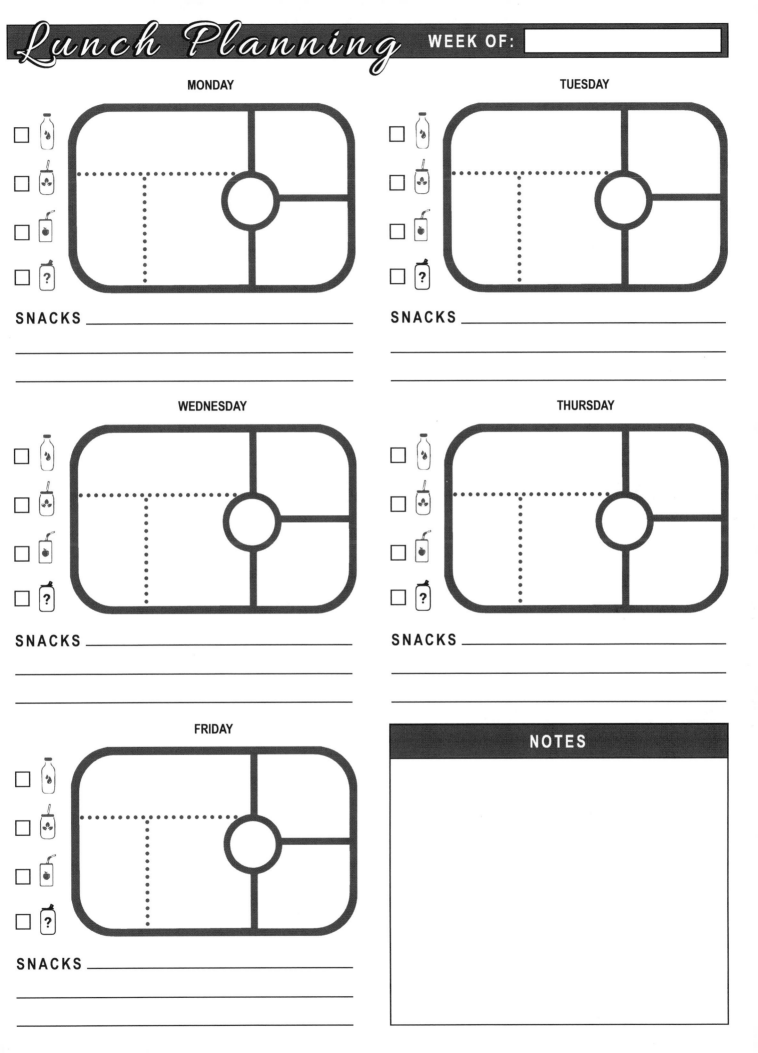

SNACKS _____

_____

_____

TUESDAY

SNACKS _____

_____

_____

WEDNESDAY

SNACKS _____

_____

_____

THURSDAY

SNACKS _____

_____

_____

FRIDAY

SNACKS _____

_____

_____

NOTES

Lunch Planning

MONDAY

☐
☐
☐
☐

SNACKS _____

_____

_____

TUESDAY

☐
☐
☐
☐

SNACKS _____

_____

_____

WEDNESDAY

☐
☐
☐
☐

SNACKS _____

_____

_____

THURSDAY

☐
☐
☐
☐

SNACKS _____

_____

_____

FRIDAY

☐
☐
☐
☐

SNACKS _____

_____

_____

NOTES

Lunch Planning

WEEK OF:

MONDAY

SNACKS _____

_____

_____

TUESDAY

SNACKS _____

_____

_____

WEDNESDAY

SNACKS _____

_____

_____

THURSDAY

SNACKS _____

_____

_____

FRIDAY

SNACKS _____

_____

_____

NOTES

Lunch Planning

MONDAY

☐
☐
☐
☐

SNACKS _____
_____
_____

TUESDAY

☐
☐
☐
☐

SNACKS _____
_____
_____

WEDNESDAY

☐
☐
☐
☐

SNACKS _____
_____
_____

THURSDAY

☐
☐
☐
☐

SNACKS _____
_____
_____

FRIDAY

☐
☐
☐
☐

SNACKS _____
_____
_____

NOTES

Lunch Planning

MONDAY

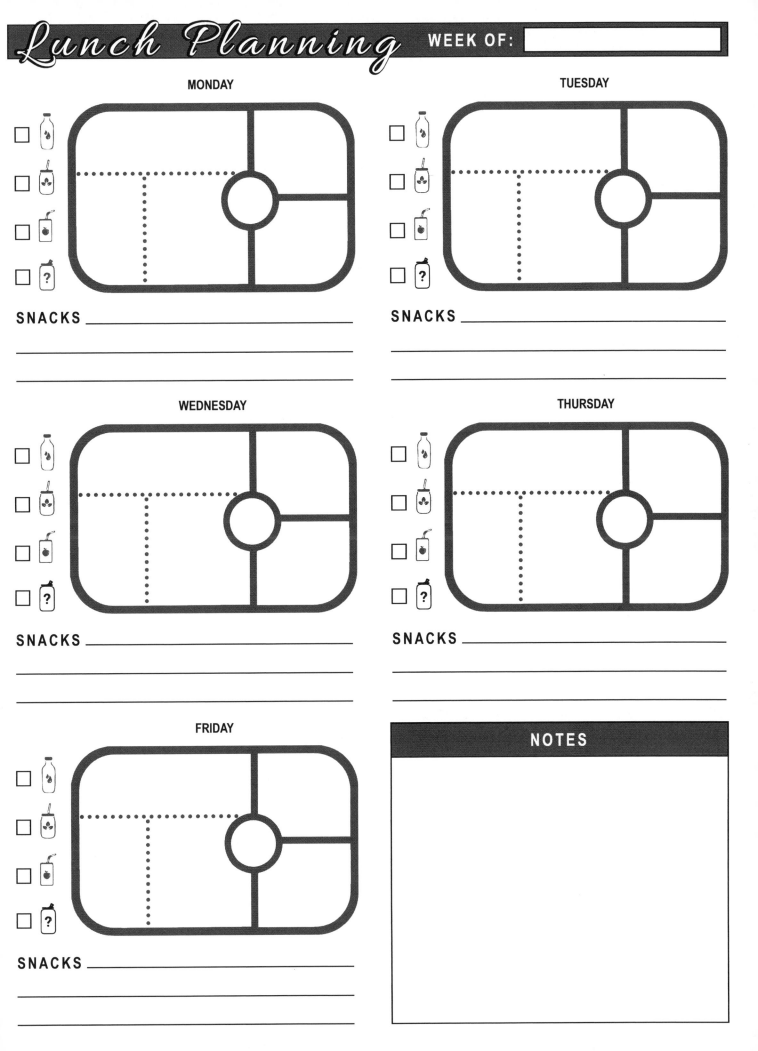

SNACKS _____

_____

_____

TUESDAY

SNACKS _____

_____

_____

WEDNESDAY

SNACKS _____

_____

_____

THURSDAY

SNACKS _____

_____

_____

FRIDAY

SNACKS _____

_____

_____

NOTES

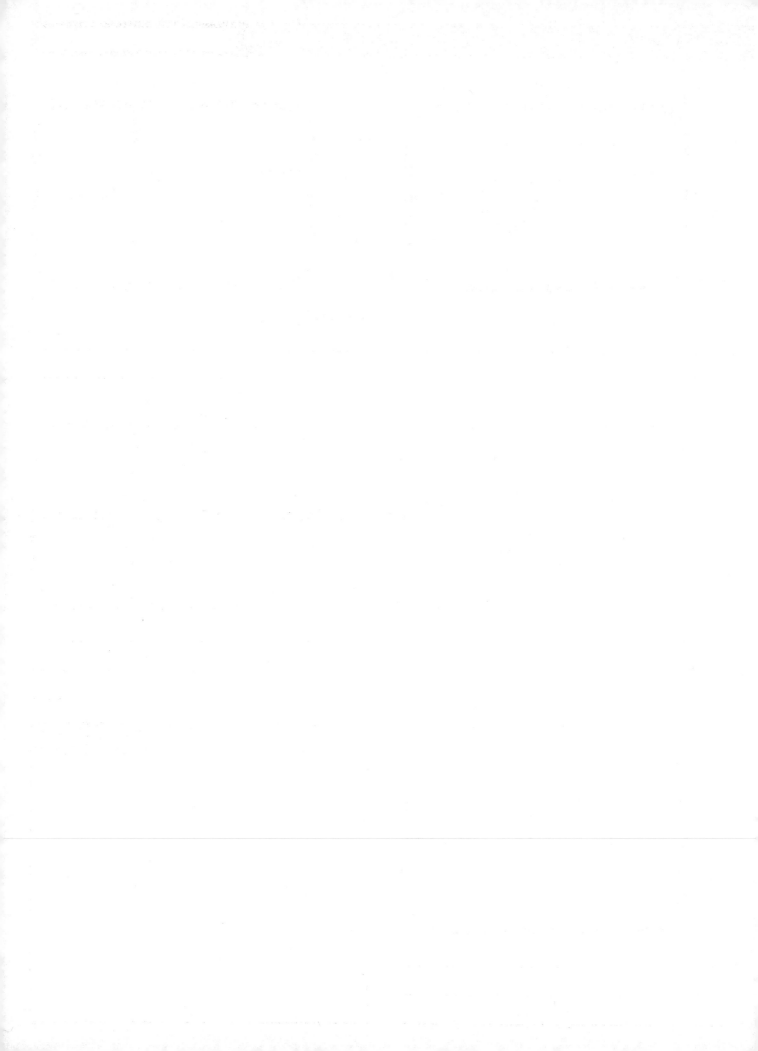

Lunch Planning

WEEK OF:

MONDAY

SNACKS _____

_____

_____

TUESDAY

SNACKS _____

_____

_____

WEDNESDAY

SNACKS _____

_____

_____

THURSDAY

SNACKS _____

_____

_____

FRIDAY

SNACKS _____

_____

_____

NOTES

Lunch Planning

MONDAY

☐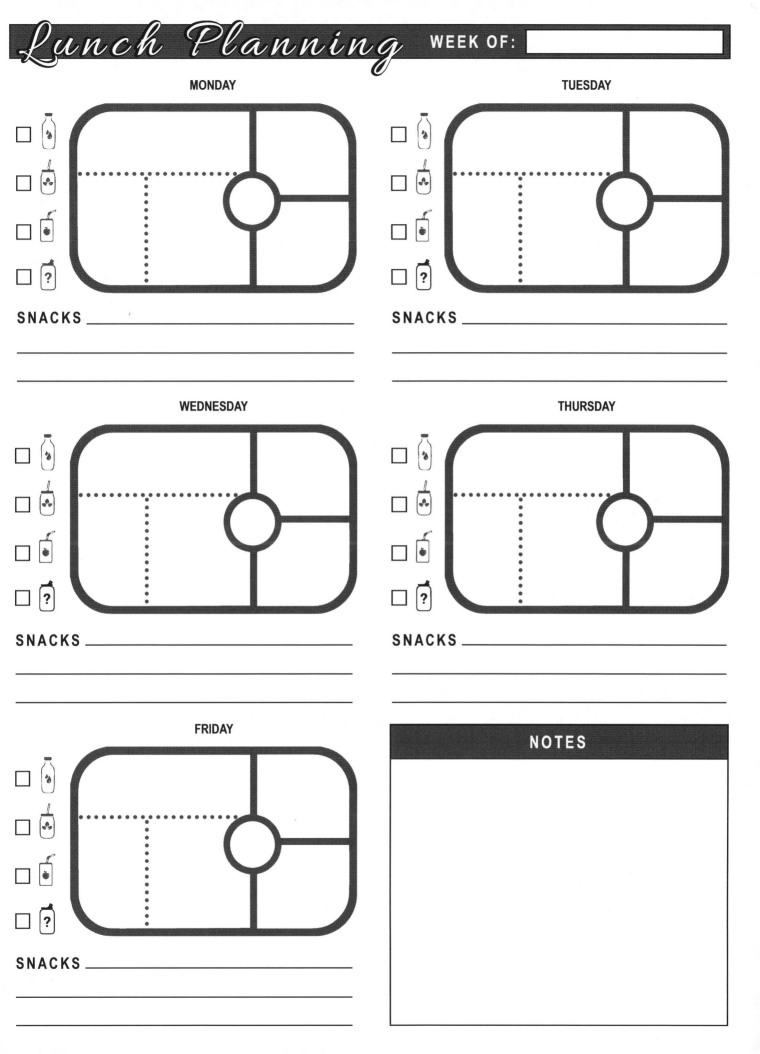
☐
☐
☐

SNACKS _____

_____

_____

TUESDAY

☐
☐
☐
☐

SNACKS _____

_____

_____

WEDNESDAY

☐
☐
☐
☐

SNACKS _____

_____

_____

THURSDAY

☐
☐
☐
☐

SNACKS _____

_____

_____

FRIDAY

☐
☐
☐
☐

SNACKS _____

_____

_____

NOTES

Lunch Planning

WEEK OF:

MONDAY

SNACKS _____

_____

_____

TUESDAY

SNACKS _____

_____

_____

WEDNESDAY

SNACKS _____

_____

_____

THURSDAY

SNACKS _____

_____

_____

FRIDAY

SNACKS _____

_____

_____

NOTES

Lunch Planning

MONDAY

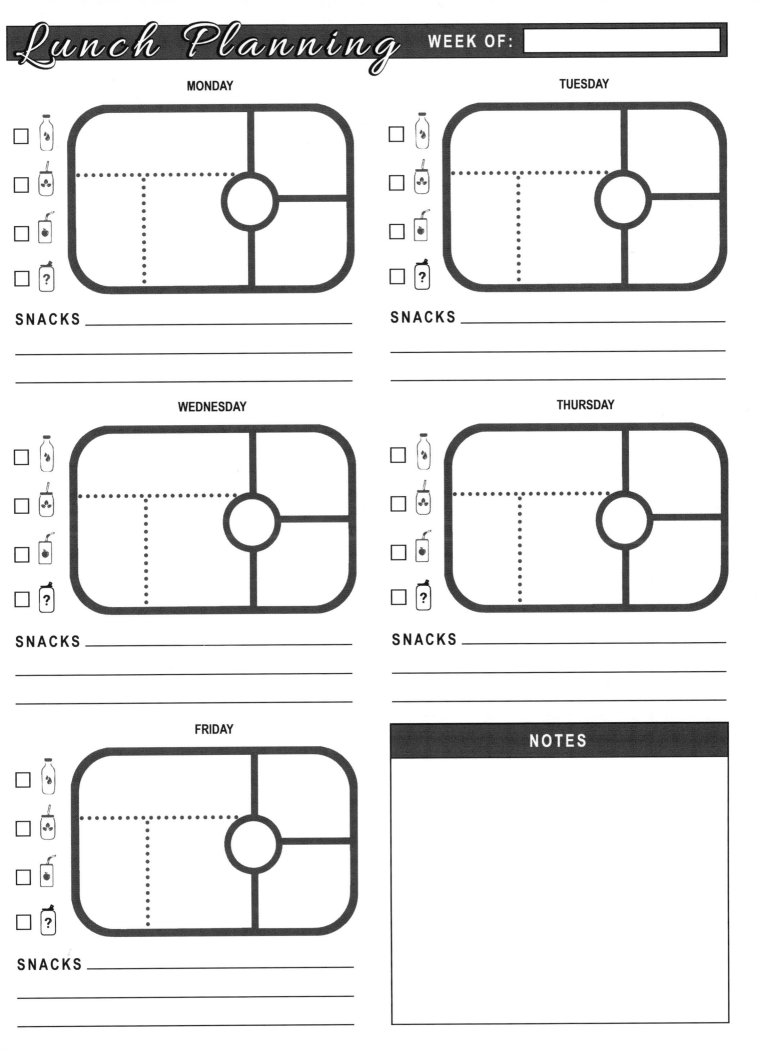

SNACKS _____

_____

_____

TUESDAY

SNACKS _____

_____

_____

WEDNESDAY

SNACKS _____

_____

_____

THURSDAY

SNACKS _____

_____

_____

FRIDAY

SNACKS _____

_____

_____

NOTES

Lunch Planning WEEK OF: [   ]

MONDAY

SNACKS _____

_____

_____

TUESDAY

SNACKS _____

_____

_____

WEDNESDAY

SNACKS _____

_____

_____

THURSDAY

SNACKS _____

_____

_____

FRIDAY

SNACKS _____

_____

_____

NOTES

Lunch Planning

WEEK OF:

MONDAY

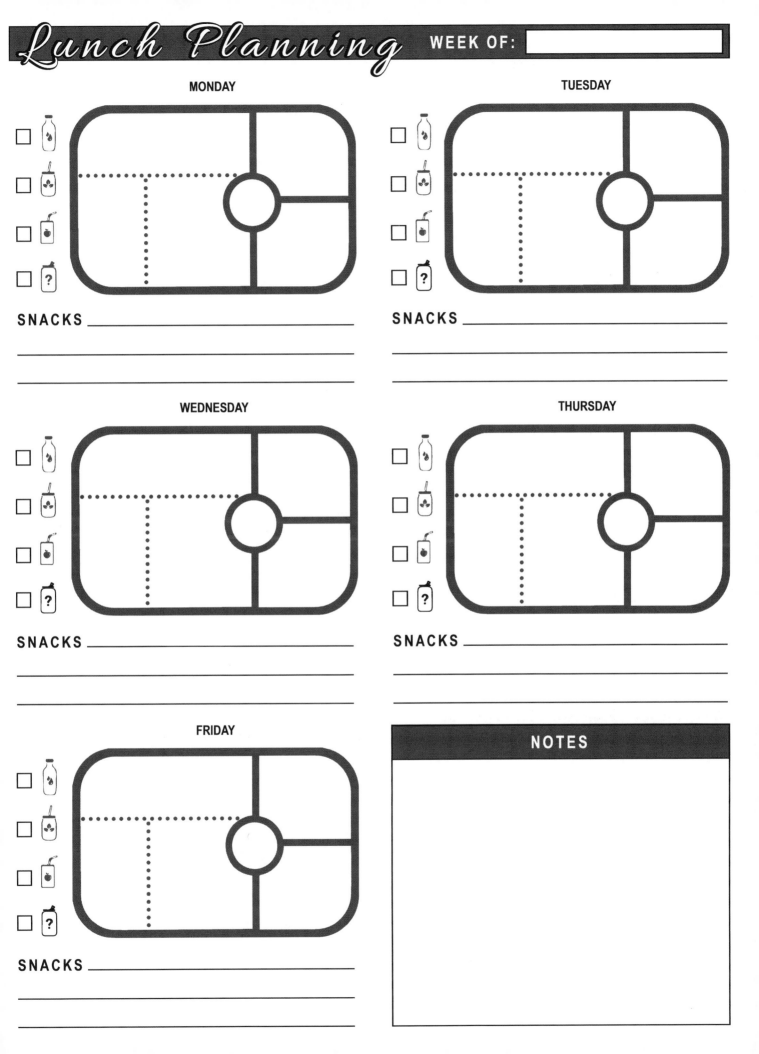

SNACKS _____

_____

_____

TUESDAY

SNACKS _____

_____

_____

WEDNESDAY

SNACKS _____

_____

_____

THURSDAY

SNACKS _____

_____

_____

FRIDAY

SNACKS _____

_____

_____

NOTES

Lunch Planning

MONDAY

SNACKS _____

_____

_____

TUESDAY

SNACKS _____

_____

_____

WEDNESDAY

SNACKS _____

_____

_____

THURSDAY

SNACKS _____

_____

_____

FRIDAY

SNACKS _____

_____

_____

NOTES

Lunch Planning

WEEK OF: _____

MONDAY

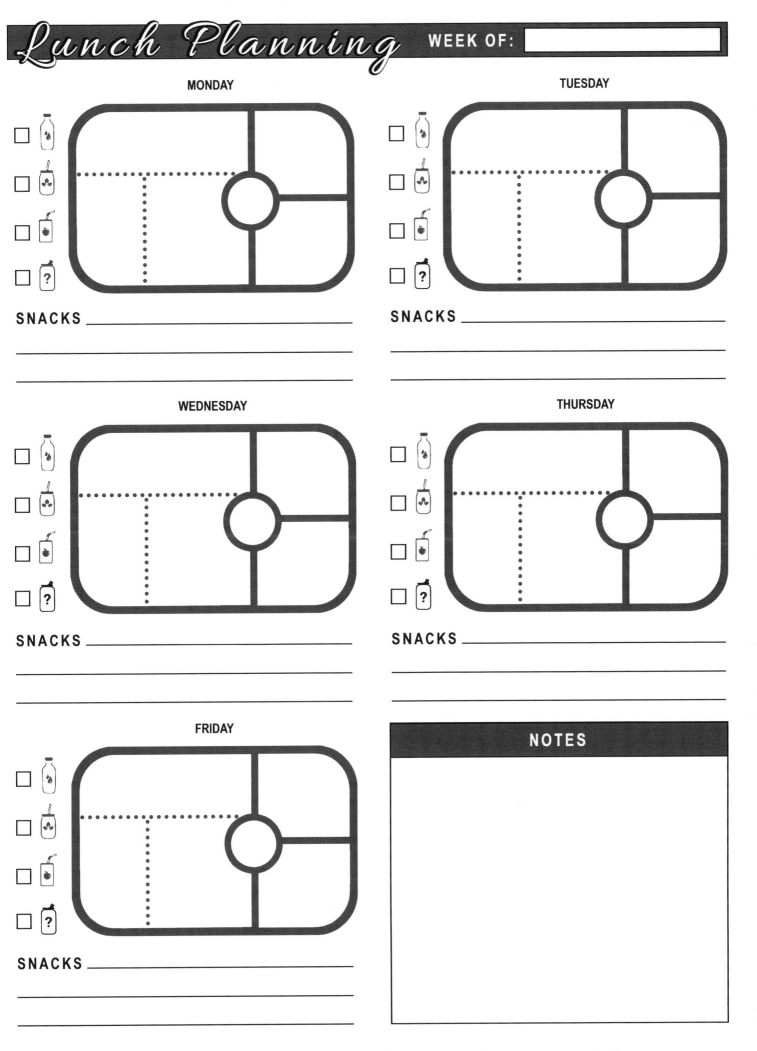

SNACKS _____

_____

_____

TUESDAY

SNACKS _____

_____

_____

WEDNESDAY

SNACKS _____

_____

_____

THURSDAY

SNACKS _____

_____

_____

FRIDAY

SNACKS _____

_____

_____

NOTES

Lunch Planning

WEEK OF:

MONDAY

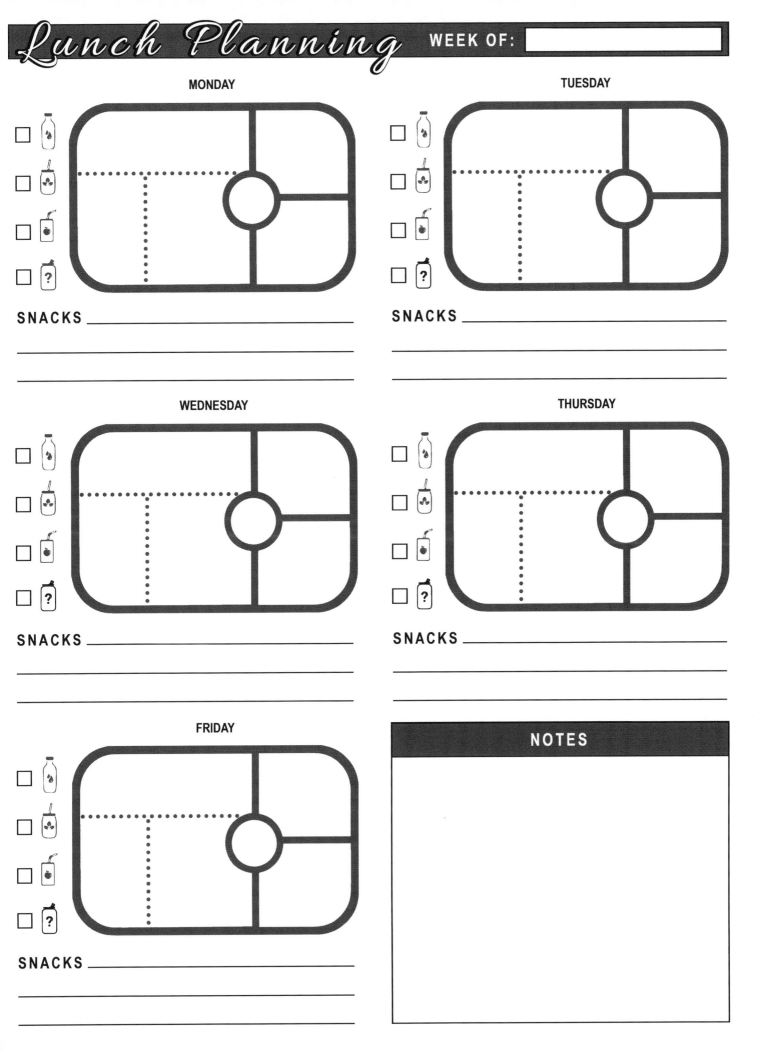

SNACKS _____

_____

_____

TUESDAY

SNACKS _____

_____

_____

WEDNESDAY

SNACKS _____

_____

_____

THURSDAY

SNACKS _____

_____

_____

FRIDAY

SNACKS _____

_____

_____

NOTES

Lunch Planning

WEEK OF:

MONDAY

SNACKS _____

_____

_____

TUESDAY

SNACKS _____

_____

_____

WEDNESDAY

SNACKS _____

_____

_____

THURSDAY

SNACKS _____

_____

_____

FRIDAY

SNACKS _____

_____

_____

NOTES

Lunch Planning

WEEK OF:

MONDAY

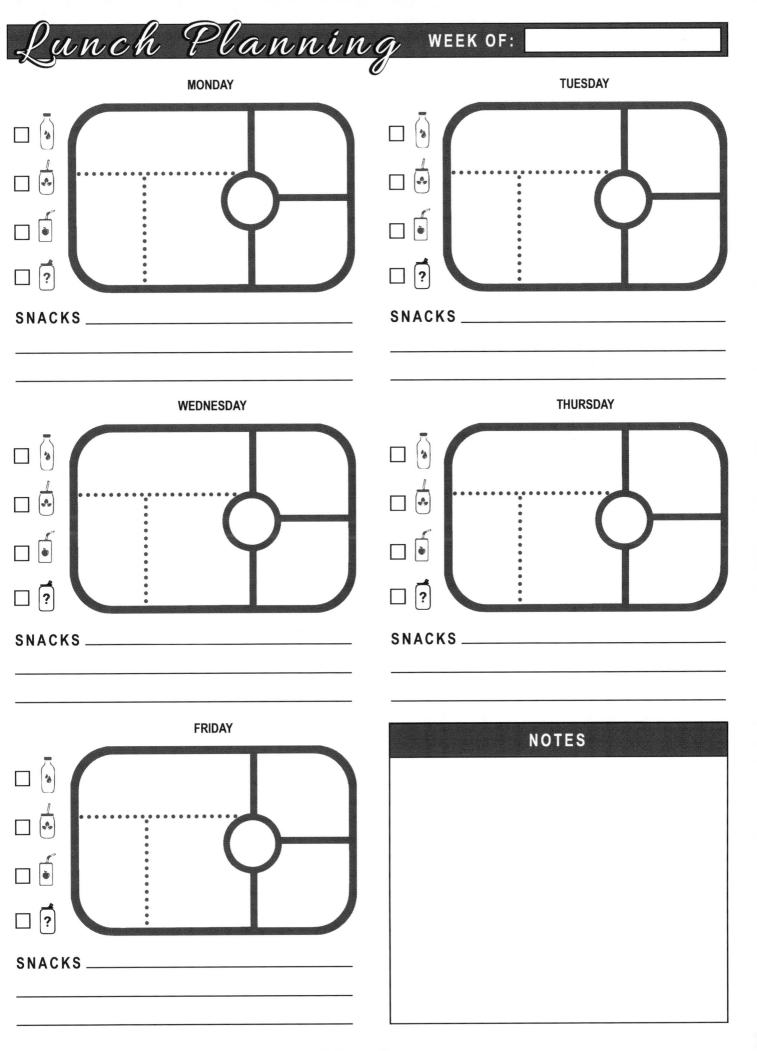

SNACKS _____

_____

_____

TUESDAY

SNACKS _____

_____

_____

WEDNESDAY

SNACKS _____

_____

_____

THURSDAY

SNACKS _____

_____

_____

FRIDAY

SNACKS _____

_____

_____

NOTES

Lunch Planning

WEEK OF:

MONDAY

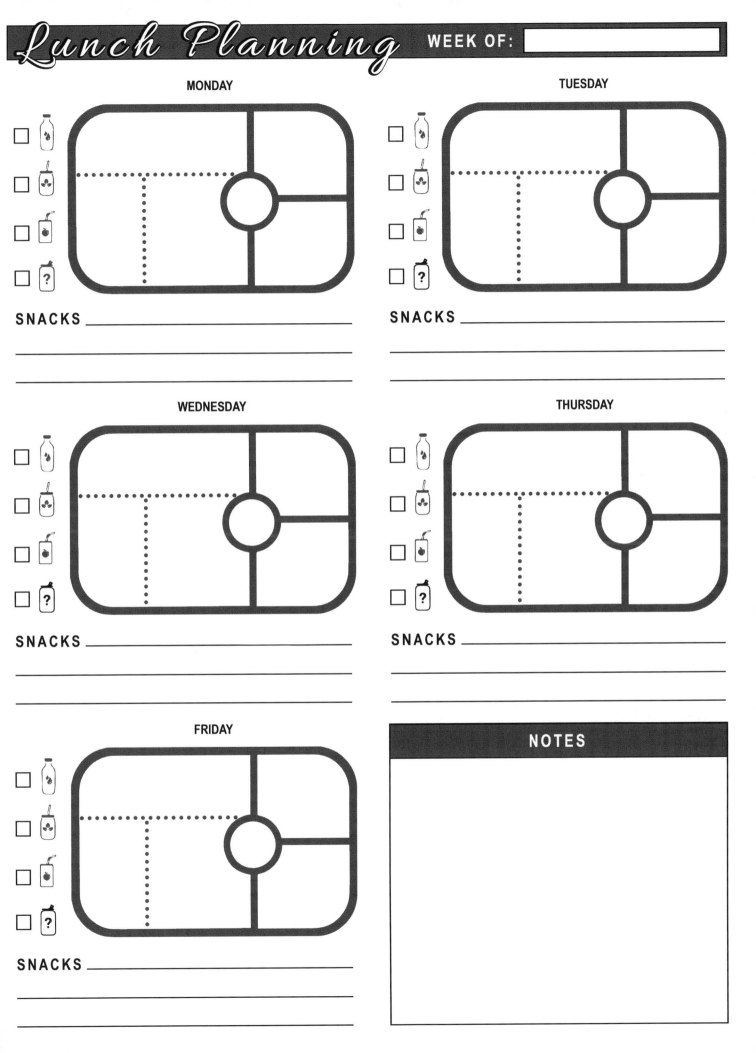

SNACKS _____

_____

_____

TUESDAY

SNACKS _____

_____

_____

WEDNESDAY

SNACKS _____

_____

_____

THURSDAY

SNACKS _____

_____

_____

FRIDAY

SNACKS _____

_____

_____

NOTES

Lunch Planning

MONDAY

☐
☐
☐
☐

SNACKS _____

_____

_____

TUESDAY

☐
☐
☐
☐

SNACKS _____

_____

_____

WEDNESDAY

☐
☐
☐
☐

SNACKS _____

_____

_____

THURSDAY

☐
☐
☐
☐

SNACKS _____

_____

_____

FRIDAY

☐
☐
☐
☐

SNACKS _____

_____

_____

NOTES

Lunch Planning

WEEK OF:

MONDAY

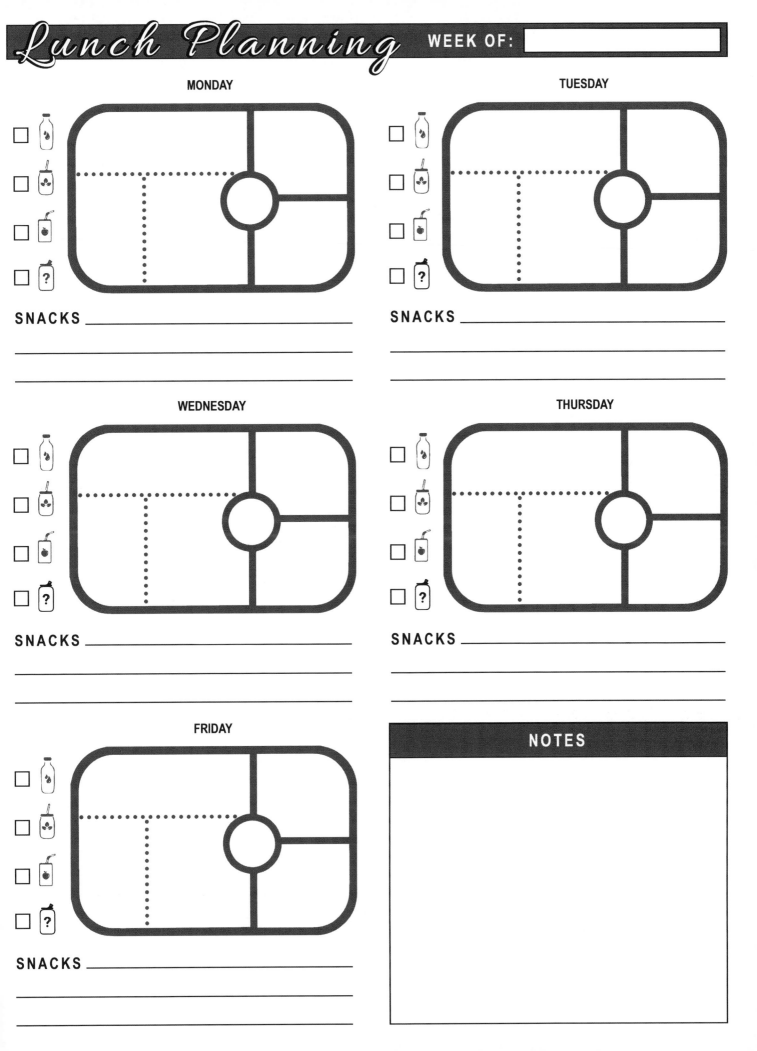

SNACKS _____

_____

_____

TUESDAY

SNACKS _____

_____

_____

WEDNESDAY

SNACKS _____

_____

_____

THURSDAY

SNACKS _____

_____

_____

FRIDAY

SNACKS _____

_____

_____

NOTES

Lunch Planning

MONDAY

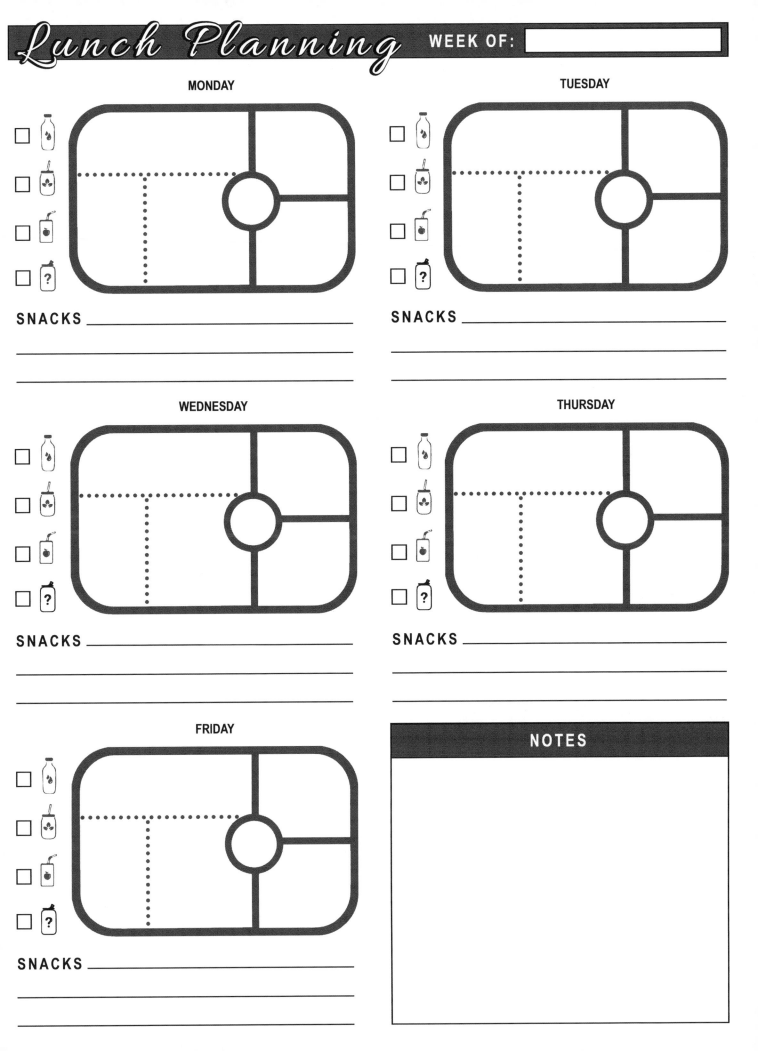

SNACKS _____

_____

_____

TUESDAY

SNACKS _____

_____

_____

WEDNESDAY

SNACKS _____

_____

_____

THURSDAY

SNACKS _____

_____

_____

FRIDAY

SNACKS _____

_____

_____

NOTES

Lunch Planning

MONDAY

☐
☐
☐
☐

SNACKS _____

_____

_____

TUESDAY

☐
☐
☐
☐

SNACKS _____

_____

_____

WEDNESDAY

☐
☐
☐
☐

SNACKS _____

_____

_____

THURSDAY

☐
☐
☐
☐

SNACKS _____

_____

_____

FRIDAY

☐
☐
☐
☐

SNACKS _____

_____

_____

NOTES

Lunch Planning

WEEK OF:

MONDAY

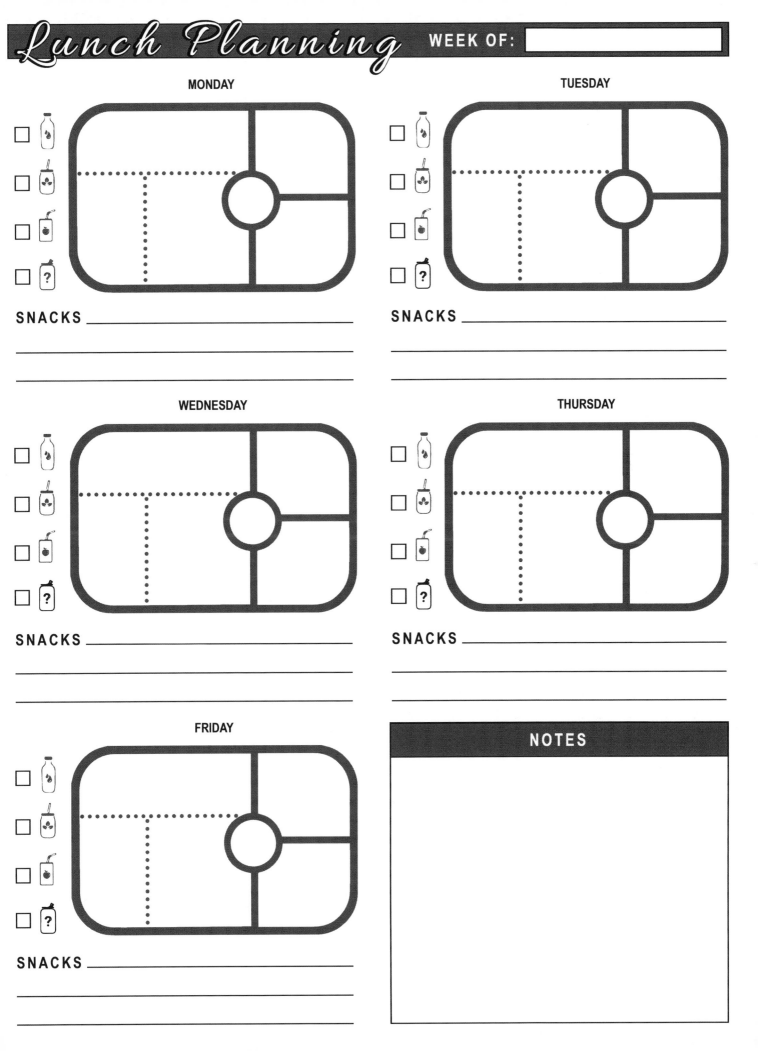

SNACKS _____

_____

_____

TUESDAY

SNACKS _____

_____

_____

WEDNESDAY

SNACKS _____

_____

_____

THURSDAY

SNACKS _____

_____

_____

FRIDAY

SNACKS _____

_____

_____

NOTES

Lunch Planning

WEEK OF:

MONDAY

☐
☐
☐
☐

SNACKS _____

_____

_____

TUESDAY

☐
☐
☐
☐

SNACKS _____

_____

_____

WEDNESDAY

☐
☐
☐
☐

SNACKS _____

_____

_____

THURSDAY

☐
☐
☐
☐

SNACKS _____

_____

_____

FRIDAY

☐
☐
☐
☐

SNACKS _____

_____

_____

NOTES

Lunch Planning

MONDAY

SNACKS _____

_____

_____

TUESDAY

SNACKS _____

_____

_____

WEDNESDAY

SNACKS _____

_____

_____

THURSDAY

SNACKS _____

_____

_____

FRIDAY

SNACKS _____

_____

_____

NOTES

Lunch Planning

WEEK OF:

MONDAY

SNACKS _____

_____

_____

TUESDAY

SNACKS _____

_____

_____

WEDNESDAY

SNACKS _____

_____

_____

THURSDAY

SNACKS _____

_____

_____

FRIDAY

SNACKS _____

_____

NOTES

Lunch Planning

MONDAY

☐
☐
☐
☐

SNACKS _____

_____

_____

TUESDAY

☐
☐
☐
☐

SNACKS _____

_____

_____

WEDNESDAY

☐
☐
☐
☐

SNACKS _____

_____

_____

THURSDAY

☐
☐
☐
☐

SNACKS _____

_____

_____

FRIDAY

☐
☐
☐
☐

SNACKS _____

_____

_____

NOTES

Lunch Planning

MONDAY

☐
☐
☐
☐

S N A C K S _____
_____
_____

TUESDAY

☐
☐
☐
☐

S N A C K S _____
_____
_____

WEDNESDAY

☐
☐
☐
☐

S N A C K S _____
_____
_____

THURSDAY

☐
☐
☐
☐

S N A C K S _____
_____
_____

FRIDAY

☐
☐
☐
☐

S N A C K S _____
_____
_____

NOTES

Lunch Planning

MONDAY

☐
☐
☐
☐

SNACKS _____

_____

_____

TUESDAY

☐
☐
☐
☐

SNACKS _____

_____

_____

WEDNESDAY

☐
☐
☐
☐

SNACKS _____

_____

_____

THURSDAY

☐
☐
☐
☐

SNACKS _____

_____

_____

FRIDAY

☐
☐
☐
☐

SNACKS _____

_____

_____

NOTES

Lunch Planning

WEEK OF:

MONDAY

SNACKS _____

_____

_____

TUESDAY

SNACKS _____

_____

_____

WEDNESDAY

SNACKS _____

_____

_____

THURSDAY

SNACKS _____

_____

_____

FRIDAY

SNACKS _____

_____

_____

NOTES

Lunch Planning

WEEK OF: _____

MONDAY

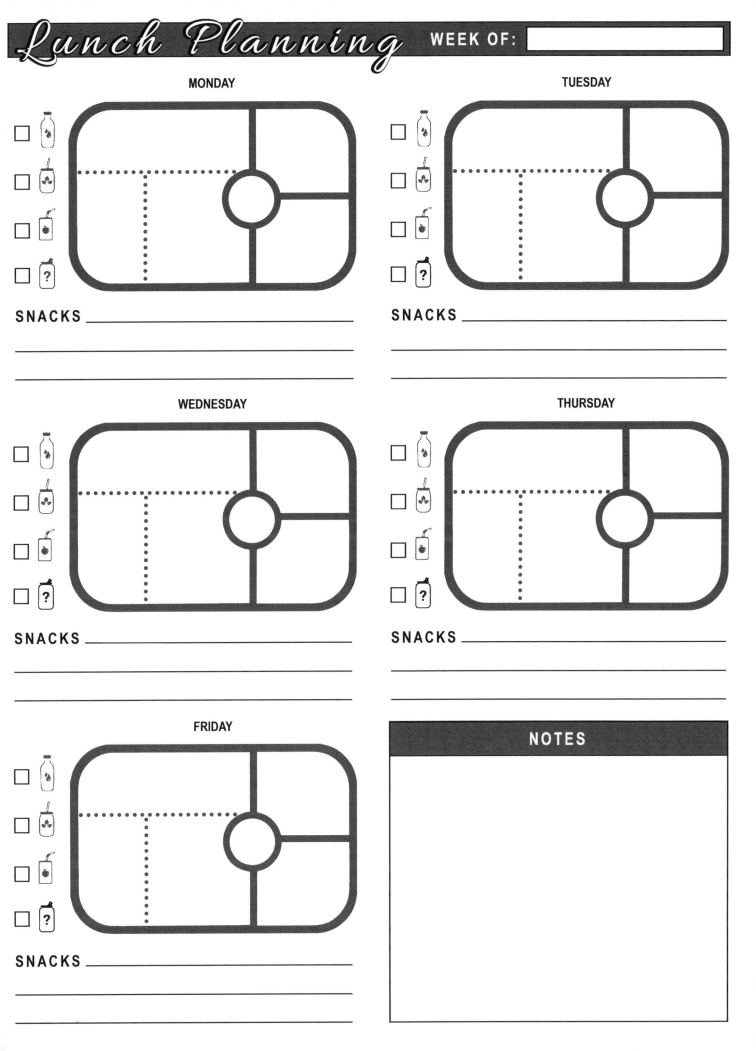

☐
☐
☐
☐

SNACKS _____

_____

_____

TUESDAY

☐
☐
☐
☐

SNACKS _____

_____

_____

WEDNESDAY

☐
☐
☐
☐

SNACKS _____

_____

_____

THURSDAY

☐
☐
☐
☐

SNACKS _____

_____

_____

FRIDAY

☐
☐
☐
☐

SNACKS _____

_____

_____

NOTES

Lunch Planning

WEEK OF:

MONDAY

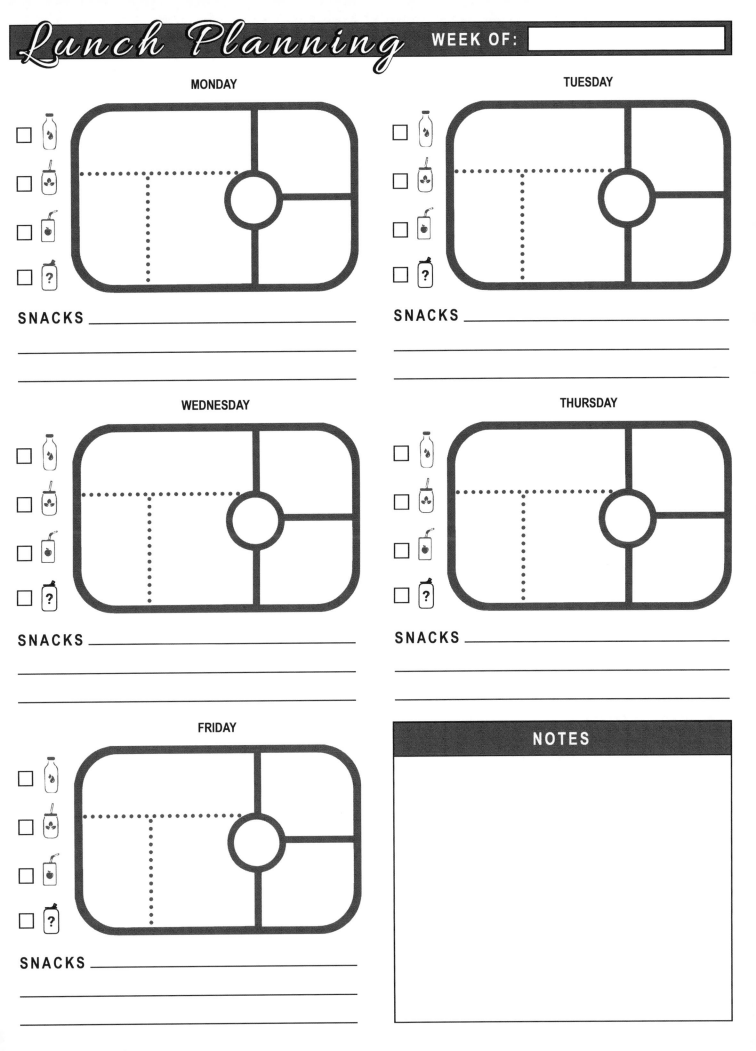

SNACKS _____

_____

_____

TUESDAY

SNACKS _____

_____

_____

WEDNESDAY

SNACKS _____

_____

_____

THURSDAY

SNACKS _____

_____

_____

FRIDAY

SNACKS _____

_____

_____

NOTES

Lunch Planning

WEEK OF:

MONDAY

SNACKS _____

_____

_____

TUESDAY

SNACKS _____

_____

_____

WEDNESDAY

SNACKS _____

_____

_____

THURSDAY

SNACKS _____

_____

_____

FRIDAY

SNACKS _____

_____

_____

NOTES

Lunch Planning

WEEK OF:

MONDAY

SNACKS _____

_____

_____

TUESDAY

SNACKS _____

_____

_____

WEDNESDAY

SNACKS _____

_____

_____

THURSDAY

SNACKS _____

_____

_____

FRIDAY

SNACKS _____

_____

_____

NOTES

Lunch Planning

WEEK OF:

MONDAY

SNACKS _____

_____

_____

TUESDAY

SNACKS _____

_____

_____

WEDNESDAY

SNACKS _____

_____

_____

THURSDAY

SNACKS _____

_____

_____

FRIDAY

SNACKS _____

_____

_____

NOTES

Lunch Planning

MONDAY

SNACKS _____

_____

_____

TUESDAY

SNACKS _____

_____

_____

WEDNESDAY

SNACKS _____

_____

_____

THURSDAY

SNACKS _____

_____

_____

FRIDAY

SNACKS _____

_____

_____

NOTES

Lunch Planning

MONDAY

☐
☐
☐
☐

SNACKS _____

_____

_____

TUESDAY

☐
☐
☐
☐

SNACKS _____

_____

_____

WEDNESDAY

☐
☐
☐
☐

SNACKS _____

_____

_____

THURSDAY

☐
☐
☐
☐

SNACKS _____

_____

_____

FRIDAY

☐
☐
☐
☐

SNACKS _____

_____

_____

NOTES

Lunch Planning

MONDAY

☐ 🍼
☐ 🥤
☐ 🧃
☐ ❓

SNACKS _____

_____

_____

TUESDAY

☐ 🍼
☐ 🥤
☐ 🧃
☐ ❓

SNACKS _____

_____

_____

WEDNESDAY

☐ 🍼
☐ 🥤
☐ 🧃
☐ ❓

SNACKS _____

_____

_____

THURSDAY

☐ 🍼
☐ 🥤
☐ 🧃
☐ ❓

SNACKS _____

_____

_____

FRIDAY

☐ 🍼
☐ 🥤
☐ 🧃
☐ ❓

SNACKS _____

_____

_____

NOTES

Lunch Planning

MONDAY

☐
☐
☐
☐

SNACKS _____

_____

_____

TUESDAY

☐
☐
☐
☐

SNACKS _____

_____

_____

WEDNESDAY

☐
☐
☐
☐

SNACKS _____

_____

_____

THURSDAY

☐
☐
☐
☐

SNACKS _____

_____

_____

FRIDAY

☐
☐
☐
☐

SNACKS _____

_____

_____

NOTES

Lunch Planning

WEEK OF:

MONDAY

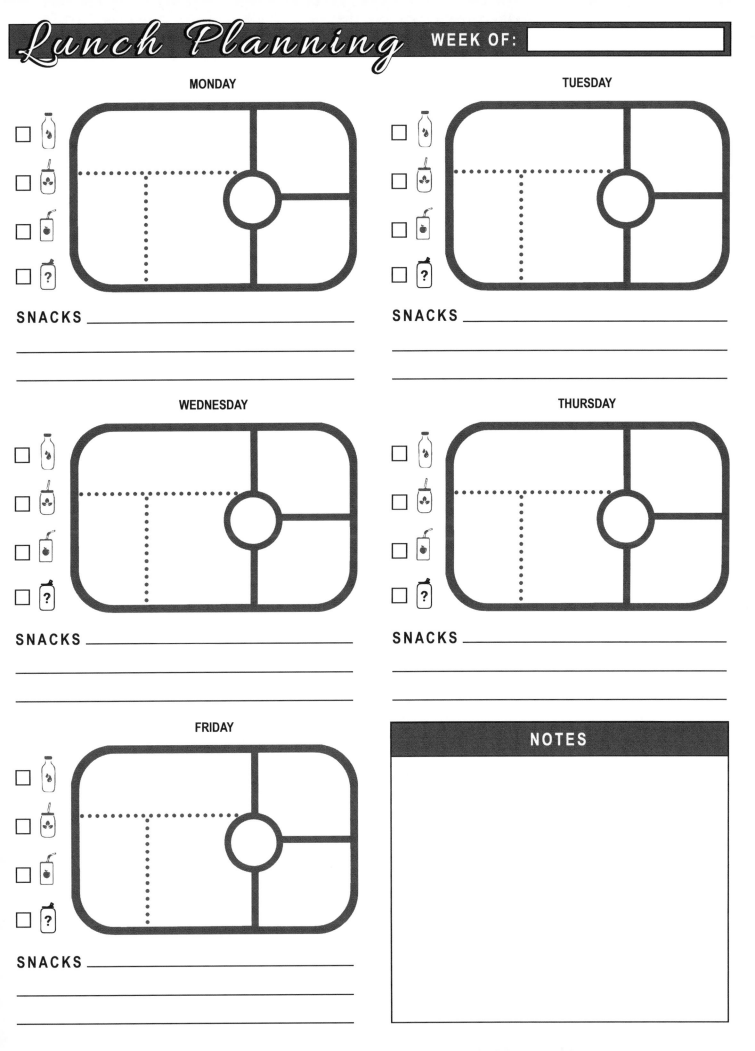

SNACKS _____

_____

_____

TUESDAY

SNACKS _____

_____

_____

WEDNESDAY

SNACKS _____

_____

_____

THURSDAY

SNACKS _____

_____

_____

FRIDAY

SNACKS _____

_____

_____

NOTES

Lunch Planning

WEEK OF:

MONDAY

SNACKS _____

_____

_____

TUESDAY

SNACKS _____

_____

_____

WEDNESDAY

SNACKS _____

_____

_____

THURSDAY

SNACKS _____

_____

_____

FRIDAY

SNACKS _____

_____

_____

NOTES

Lunch Planning

MONDAY

☐
☐
☐
☐

SNACKS _____

_____

_____

TUESDAY

☐
☐
☐
☐

SNACKS _____

_____

_____

WEDNESDAY

☐
☐
☐
☐

SNACKS _____

_____

_____

THURSDAY

☐
☐
☐
☐

SNACKS _____

_____

_____

FRIDAY

☐
☐
☐
☐

SNACKS _____

_____

_____

NOTES

Lunch Planning

WEEK OF: _____

MONDAY

SNACKS _____
_____
_____

TUESDAY

SNACKS _____
_____
_____

WEDNESDAY

SNACKS _____
_____
_____

THURSDAY

SNACKS _____
_____
_____

FRIDAY

SNACKS _____
_____
_____

NOTES

Lunch Planning

MONDAY

SNACKS _____

_____

_____

TUESDAY

SNACKS _____

_____

_____

WEDNESDAY

SNACKS _____

_____

_____

THURSDAY

SNACKS _____

_____

_____

FRIDAY

SNACKS _____

_____

_____

NOTES

Lunch Planning

WEEK OF:

MONDAY

☐
☐
☐
☐

SNACKS _____

_____

_____

TUESDAY

☐
☐
☐
☐

SNACKS _____

_____

_____

WEDNESDAY

☐
☐
☐
☐

SNACKS _____

_____

_____

THURSDAY

☐
☐
☐
☐

SNACKS _____

_____

_____

FRIDAY

☐
☐
☐
☐

SNACKS _____

_____

_____

NOTES

Lunch Planning

MONDAY

SNACKS _____

_____

_____

TUESDAY

SNACKS _____

_____

_____

WEDNESDAY

SNACKS _____

_____

_____

THURSDAY

SNACKS _____

_____

_____

FRIDAY

SNACKS _____

_____

_____

NOTES

Lunch Planning

MONDAY

☐ ☐ ☐ ☐

SNACKS _____

_____

_____

TUESDAY

☐ ☐ ☐ ☐

SNACKS _____

_____

_____

WEDNESDAY

☐ ☐ ☐ ☐

SNACKS _____

_____

_____

THURSDAY

☐ ☐ ☐ ☐

SNACKS _____

_____

_____

FRIDAY

☐ ☐ ☐ ☐

SNACKS _____

_____

_____

NOTES

Lunch Planning

WEEK OF:

MONDAY

SNACKS _____

_____

_____

TUESDAY

SNACKS _____

_____

_____

WEDNESDAY

SNACKS _____

_____

_____

THURSDAY

SNACKS _____

_____

_____

FRIDAY

SNACKS _____

_____

_____

NOTES

Lunch Planning

WEEK OF:

MONDAY

SNACKS _____

_____

_____

TUESDAY

SNACKS _____

_____

_____

WEDNESDAY

SNACKS _____

_____

_____

THURSDAY

SNACKS _____

_____

_____

FRIDAY

SNACKS _____

_____

_____

NOTES

Lunch Planning

WEEK OF:

MONDAY

SNACKS _____

_____

_____

TUESDAY

SNACKS _____

_____

_____

WEDNESDAY

SNACKS _____

_____

_____

THURSDAY

SNACKS _____

_____

_____

FRIDAY

SNACKS _____

_____

_____

NOTES

Lunch Planning

WEEK OF:

MONDAY

SNACKS _____

_____

_____

TUESDAY

SNACKS _____

_____

_____

WEDNESDAY

SNACKS _____

_____

_____

THURSDAY

SNACKS _____

_____

_____

FRIDAY

SNACKS _____

_____

_____

NOTES

Lunch Planning

WEEK OF:

MONDAY

SNACKS _____

_____

_____

TUESDAY

SNACKS _____

_____

_____

WEDNESDAY

SNACKS _____

_____

_____

THURSDAY

SNACKS _____

_____

_____

FRIDAY

SNACKS _____

_____

_____

NOTES

Lunch Planning

WEEK OF:

MONDAY

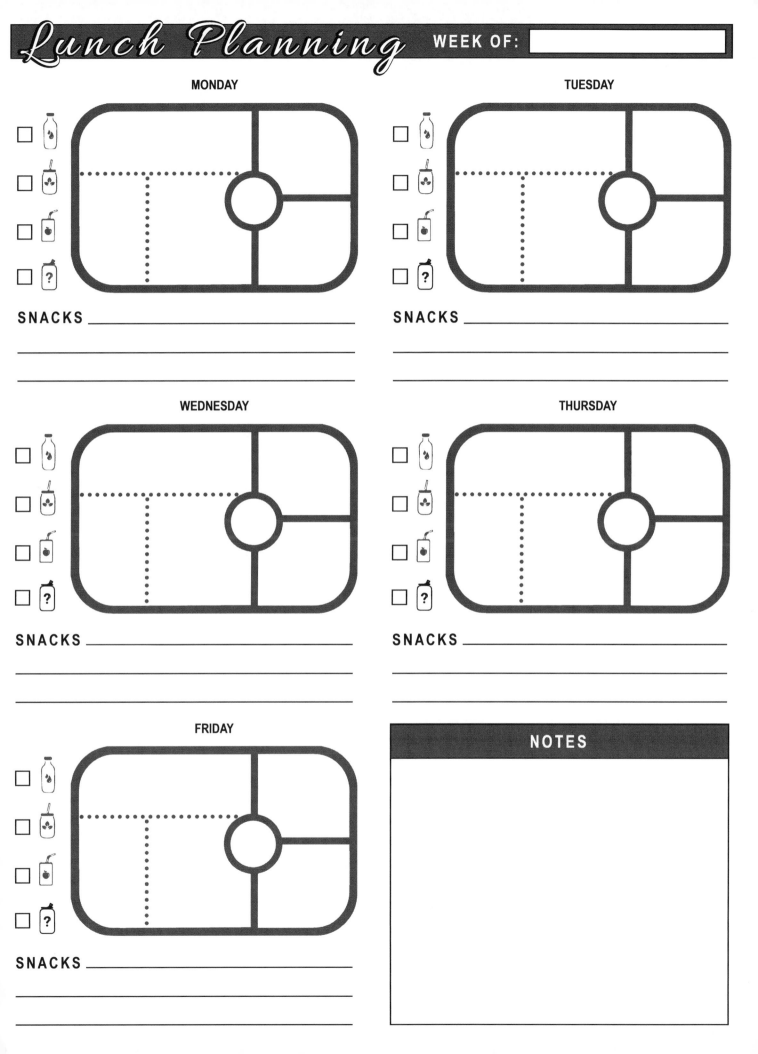

SNACKS _____

_____

_____

TUESDAY

SNACKS _____

_____

_____

WEDNESDAY

SNACKS _____

_____

_____

THURSDAY

SNACKS _____

_____

_____

FRIDAY

SNACKS _____

_____

_____

NOTES

Lunch Planning

WEEK OF:

MONDAY

SNACKS _____

_____

_____

TUESDAY

SNACKS _____

_____

_____

WEDNESDAY

SNACKS _____

_____

_____

THURSDAY

SNACKS _____

_____

_____

FRIDAY

SNACKS _____

_____

_____

NOTES

Lunch Planning

MONDAY

☐ ☐ ☐ ☐

SNACKS _____

_____

_____

TUESDAY

☐ ☐ ☐ ☐

SNACKS _____

_____

_____

WEDNESDAY

☐ ☐ ☐ ☐

SNACKS _____

_____

_____

THURSDAY

☐ ☐ ☐ ☐

SNACKS _____

_____

_____

FRIDAY

☐ ☐ ☐ ☐

SNACKS _____

_____

_____

NOTES

LOVE IT   ✓ LIKE IT   (?) NEVER TRIED IT   😐 DON'T REALLY LIKE IT   ✗ HATE IT

LOVE IT   LIKE IT   NEVER TRIED IT   DON'T REALLY LIKE IT   HATE IT

LOVE IT   ✓ LIKE IT   ? NEVER TRIED IT   😐 DON'T REALLY LIKE IT   ✗ HATE IT

Lunch Notes